The International Behavioural an

REFLECTIONS ON THE NUDE

TAVISTOCK

The International Behavioural and Social Sciences Library

PSYCHOLOGY OF ART: SELECTED WORKS OF
ADRIAN STOKES
In 6 Volumes

REFLECTIONS ON THE NUDE

ADRIAN STOKES

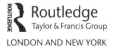

Routledge
Taylor & Francis Group
LONDON AND NEW YORK

First published in 1967 by
Tavistock Publications Limited

Reprinted in 2001 by
Routledge
2 Park Square, Milton Park, Abingdon, Oxon, OX14 4RN

Simultaneously published in the USA and Canada by Routledge

711 Third Avenue, New York, NY 10017

Transferred to Digital Printing 2007

Routledge is an imprint of the Taylor & Francis Group

First issued in paperback 2013

The publishers have made every effort to contact authors/copyright holders
of the works reprinted in the *International Behavioural and Social Sciences
Library*. This has not been possible in every case, however, and we would
welcome correspondence from those individuals/companies we have been
unable to trace.

These reprints are taken from original copies of each book. In many cases
the condition of these originals is not perfect. The publisher has gone to
great lengths to ensure the quality of these reprints, but wishes to point
out that certain characteristics of the original copies will, of necessity, be
apparent in reprints thereof.

British Library Cataloguing in Publication Data
A CIP catalogue record for this book
is available from the British Library

Reflections on the Nude
ISBN 978-0-415-26492-1 (hbk)
ISBN 978-0-415-86600-2 (pbk)

ADRIAN STOKES

Reflections on the Nude

TAVISTOCK PUBLICATIONS

LONDON · NEW YORK · SYDNEY · TORONTO · WELLINGTON

First published in 1967
by Tavistock Publications Limited
2 Park Square, Milton Park,
Abingdon, Oxon, OX14 4RN
in 11 point Times Roman
by T. H. Brickell & Son Ltd
Gillingham, Dorset

Contents

Author's Note

The brevity of *Reflections on the Nude* is the first reason for the appearance of the lecture that follows. Although the two are not directly connected, there will be found in the lecture—written earlier—variants of the essay's argument that are now tinged, it seems, with a contrasting and conversational tone. For the first time in the volume paintings are examined singly.

Acknowledgements are due to the Editor of the *British Journal of Aesthetics* in respect of the lecture and to the Editors of *Art and Literature*, published in Paris, in respect of the original draft of the first chapter.

REFLECTIONS ON THE NUDE

I. Reflections on the Nude

Vis-à-vis the objects both of the outside world and of the inner world it is rewarding that psycho-analysis distinguishes two kinds of fundamental relationship; yet one of these relationships can be constructed at the expense of, or more usually in addition to, the other form of communion. The two modes are the part-object and the whole-object relationships. The infant's first relationships are with part-objects only, that is to say with objects that are not felt in their own nature to be foreign and altogether separate from himself. The mother's breast and his own stool are primary part-objects, the entire and separate and self-sufficient mother the primary whole-object from whose self-inclusiveness there evolves the realization of the outside world of objects as such, whatever their special functions for the perceiver and although he continues, howbeit to a lesser degree, intruding projections into them, an activity that underlies part-object relationship. Not a philosopher, as was Berkeley, the infant is able in normal development to give ground on the question whether there is an outside world which is real, that is to say, separate at least, if not yet indifferent in some contexts to his own activities. But it will have been no more true of Bishop Berkeley than of other human beings that the object conceived as a whole-object may still be treated emotionally more as a part-object.

The tendency to treat whole-objects at the same time as part-objects is very strong. It involves a degree of merging with, or being enveloped by, the object. In view of the ceaseless projective and introjective processes by which we apprehend, control, and learn, it appears extraordinary that a

3

comprehensive emotional admission of whole-object configurations is attained even fitfully.

On the other hand self-preservation will demand a recognition that the outside world is indeed disjoined, concrete; moreover the infant's growing integration depends on separateness from it. The infant's progression from the paranoid-schizoid position to the depressive, to the feelings, for instance, of loss, guilt, and responsibility rather than of persecution, is bound up with the full admission of self-contained objects in the outside world, in the first instance of the whole mother herself. The relationships to other people and to things of all kinds will partake, if only by contrast, of the relationships to her.

This must be the seemingly heartless opening to some reflections stimulated by an aspect of the nude. While the nude is by no means the whole-object prototype, it can provide imaginative translation of that prototype. Yet the word 'nude' will seem harsh to many when it does not suggest nakedness only.

We cannot discover in our own bodies the nude entirety. Narcissistic sensitivity obscures contemplation. Sex-organs often continue to be viewed as part-objects unintegrated with the tenor of the body; appendages of a temper and need averted from the delicate interaction within the organism, even to the extent of the body being conceived as an attribute of the organ, an attribution that does not dominate at least the conception of the nude, which is here thought of as enduring figuration (though the object of many intense passions) and as identical with the object that was for long the object _par excellence_ for art students.

But if the nude in this sense is a somewhat rarefied conception, it remains an immense power. The human body thus conceived is a promise of sanity. Throughout history the totality of the nude may rarely have shone, yet the potential power will have made itself deeply felt. I propose that the respect thus founded for the general body is the seal upon our respect for other human beings as such (and even for consistently objective attitudes to things as such); an important factor, therefore, in regard not only to respect but to tolerance and benevolence.

As well as for basic drives the world of objects is the setting for our projective, introjective, and splitting processes. These processes do not of themselves in many instances give rise to tolerance and respect for the objects employed. On the other hand the self-sufficiency where it is allowed to the nude, who may be the target of intense sexuality also as an independent object, accompanies our own integration or totality, our own integration of drives and character-traits. The respect for self-sufficient objects is the extension of self-respect. From this brotherhood, as it were, of the potential nude the fellow-feeling can extend at least contemplatively to every variety of psychical construction however misguided or inadequate.

It was more difficult in the past when the world was full of utter strangers, particularly in regard to their values, to culture, or to one class in contrast with another. If we are now on the way to a multi-racial culture it is partly because no custom, no ritual, no thought nor act is as incomprehensible, as distant from ourselves. Those with whom we can initially somewhat identify have multiplied even while we use them, as they have always been used, for projective purposes.

Such broad identification is the result of contact not with an aspect that a person presents to us but with the idea of his wholeness or potential wholeness since he is an inheritor, however far removed, of the mother who originally evoked our solicitude, our anxiety, as a precious whole-object that could be lost and destroyed for ever. Thus the fellow human being is by definition a whole-object who may command initially—of course it is only initially—a degree of our solicitude. This is, however, a very important adjunct of humane attitudes. Whereas there are many closer forms of identification, none of them applies this to the stranger *qua* stranger to whom in his capacity as a human being we are likely today to be most polite not only for atavistic reasons. This tie we have with him will probably lessen as we get to know him since he now looms very largely as a series of attitudes and aptitudes and certainly as the object of our projections which may be negative. We may then translate him in addition into a part-object, the possessor of some trait or function the over-riding emphasis of which becomes almost a fetish. It is as if we had entered a party, joined a conglomeration of heads and straining faces, ours among them, a succession of presences and absences with which we are compounded, that advance in answer to our call but do not always as easily retreat. Yet this merging with an object is often the tritest form of intimacy though at other times the mode of deepest sympathy and of capitulation or control.

Our constant projection and introjection tend to increase, I have indicated, the part-object aspect of relationship; not however exclusively, since in the majority of adult contacts we have already acknowledged as whole-objects, that is to say in feeling no less than in conscious judgement, what we may also treat as part-objects. The dramatic example, once more, is the temperate artist painting the nude, an act still preserved in at least some rooms of art schools. All endeavour should be to contemplate this object as entire, together with the surroundings. The face and head are but part of the body for that contemplative work in which we do not seek to reduce the form to the terms of mouth or eye, to the terms of a single function. I myself prefer the model to be, to remain, a stranger. One will consult her comfort but not the concerns that are less immediate She is an entire presence engaging the allegiance produced in the act of drawing. Artists sometimes harbour a love or brotherhood that binds them to strangers in the light of their mere presence (whereas other people tend

6

to provide at once for strangers a narrower context, however mistaken). Nevertheless aesthetic construction itself entails an envelopment also in the re-creation of a whole-object. I have called this aspect the component of invitation, the invitation to merge with the object [1].

How hard it is, then, particularly in social life to amplify the realization of whole-objects that we try to sustain. Indeed it often appears that we best foster a contact with whole-objects from a distance. Hence a perennial attraction of spectacles, of the theatre, of games, of all happenings in which people speak with their bodies as well as with their mouths. In such experiences if we ignore the crowd we can strengthen the norm of adult relationship with fellows and with Nature. And if it is difficult to value our neighbours for their wholeness, we may be able nevertheless to personalize the hive to which we belong. Further, we keep and constantly observe domestic animals who live out their lives as complicated bodies from nose to tail. The domestic animal, though not the pet, is an antithesis to the face and voice of the crowd. A crowd is no more than one fibre of a person who will never be constructed.

I do not mean to deny that face or head is by far the most expressive attribute of a person; expressive, that is, of the whole person. This succinct documentation, however, of wear and tear or of their absence may cause us to overlook the even circulation that animates a complicated structure.

Possibly the nakedness of some primitive peoples will have strengthened their grip upon sanity even though their nudity will have dramatized an extreme part-object attitude to conceptions contrasting with the whole body, namely the mask, the ceremonial face, together with a figuring forth of Spirit or Mana and the ghosts of the dead. A construction of whole-objects in primitive art has force but not a pre-eminent force. Whereas the wrapped, muffled Eskimo, deprived of nakedness, has probably been in worse case, the deformation of the body and its camouflaging fragmentation by painting and tattooing on the part of naked tribes have shown that a posesssion of the nude epitome of whole-objects has largely been gratuitous; a possession to be minimized. Of course clothes redress the balance since they are apt to dramatize the body's contours. However, as Greek art and Greek Olympiads suggest, a conception of the undivided nude is an unique attainment of tremendous import.

We realize insufficiently how rare have been potent symbols of whole-objects outside art and science and constructiveness in general. The history of ordinary building is a saga of tomb-womb-house [2]. Another part-object, the good breast, is the common fount of all that is good. But without a concomitant development of the good breast into the good whole-object we cannot be at home in an adult world: we cannot discern sufficiently between ourselves and objects nor feel the respect and brotherhood of which I have spoken with the stranger.

Where there is no call for fear or envy or the projection of hate—even today this must be a rare situation—the usage, I repeat, of extreme politeness to the stranger is a tribute to the whole-object model. Such goodwill, of course, is no guarantee of true fellowship: it often evaporates upon any intimacy, as if we were discovering that this self-sufficient entity, though entire, is not the prime whole-object, not the mother from whom we derived the good breast. Any communication with the stranger can dim even this connection; we no longer have on our hands the embodiment only of an entire human being but sectional demands and compulsions, his and our own. But I submit that the side-tracking emphases of intimacy are happiest if that first impersonal love for the whole figure at the root of respect has not been completely overborne. I call this love impersonal not because it did not arise with one person, not because it is not principally lavished still, let us hope, upon one person and one family, but because it can extend also to each individual initially, to animals, to the forms of Nature, and the artifacts of man.

I have suggested that much wider fellowship is today a possibility. I want to emphasize also a turning away from an impression of whole-objects associated with our urban environment which will soon be much expanded. By 1990, it is said, half of the greatly increased population of the world will live in conurbations of 100,000 or more, another prognostication arising from a technological development that has become a riotous growth incognisant at its root of the human needs that nourish it. The outlook for the daily spectacle of perfected whole-objects is bad. An envelopment with objects by means of predominantly part-object phantasies has for most of us ever-fresh lavish provocations, particularly in the use and guidance of machines. I won't recall instances of which I have written elsewhere that are characteristic of the scene [1]. In the past—to mention one detail—physical expenditure in craft and manual work more frequently reinforced the impression of physique: likewise the common modes of travel. As far as concerns the spectator, much work has lost in dignity, though from the point of view of the operator, of course, the constructiveness belonging to any work that has not become automatic entails the figuring forth, the repairing, of whole-objects. In this connection I have referred already to public spectacles and to the theatre; but I do not think that cinema and television should be added, largely dream-screens, poor in spatial volume and embodiment, media that contrast with sound radio wherein we may reconstruct the person at the instance of the voice, a form of recapitulation in which we have been practised since the time when from cot or pen we heard the mother who was out of sight. The case is often similar for reading.

Where there is sanity, the progression to whole-object apprehension will have been accomplished and to some degree emotionally sustained. I am discussing encouragements only

9

towards regression, exterior inducements that attach themselves to regressive tendencies in adulthood. It is a matter
whose influence we cannot calculate. But surely we admit that
the figuring forth of whole-object relationships in spheres
wider than the home or social life has a likely impress on the
quality of contact in those narrower and more primary spheres.
I therefore find it disturbing that we have constructed an urban environment the character of whose undertones does not
feed back to us the plain symbols of sanity; the configuration
of whose objects has no emphasis for the observer upon their
wholeness. The immense reduplication of our appliances, such
as switches, denotes harsh nipples instantly presented when
they are working, a chaotic pattern of commas when they are
not; unrelated alternations of the good and bad breast, the
earliest homework of splitting and projection. The machine's
power is vulgar, in tune with the most infantile phantasies,
without prudent reference to human physique. Will personal
relationships intensify among disjected pleasures, among the
harmless drugs that induce regression, and amid a mere relic
of the use of limbs?

Certainly the future will need societies devoted to the contemplation of whole-objects. Hence an ever growing importance of art. But aesthetic creativeness functions in the terms
of the environment. An artist's work can give the spectator
cause to be more at home with himself just as he, the artist,
has become more at home with himself within the surrounding environment as a result of his work. In the long run he
needs to envisage his environment as the prolonged scene of
indubitable whole-objects in correspondence with the self-
sufficiency of his artifact, however enveloping its theme. No
one can have the slightest idea what will happen to art in the
future. There must be danger that it cedes importance to hal-
lucinations induced by drugs. We have already experienced
from art a great deal of anti-art in the sense of anti-whole-
object themes, in the sense of everything-on-a-par following

10

the breakdown of distinctions, in the sense of a hypnotic envelopment by part-objects. I saw lately a huge plastic thumb, a mechanical enlargement of a cast of the artist's own thumb. (The fact that I judge it to be an original and even beautiful work is not to the point here.) The Canadian writer, Marshall McLuhan, 'has spoken'—I quote Karl Miller—'of the eclipse of the Gutenberg Galaxy, of the poor old printed word, ushering in the electronic age with its images and media, and the space age with its still stronger devices' [3].

For the many people who cannot altogether sustain satisfactory whole-object relationships it will become ever easier to embrace, or with a reverse of emotion to reject, the universe. Symbiosis can be employed to obscure both the intrinsic self and its object, to whirl them together in a manic hum. This brings me back to sound, to modern sound. What chance have we in cities today to reconstruct the whole mother from her voice? Here in London in the Burlington Arcade one can attend to people who stand and converse amid leisurely sounds of other people walking. A variety of echoes come back from the walls. It seems to me a measure of our plight that such an experience is a luxury to be treasured; apparently a haven from unending explosions of traffic that uncover no space, no amenable distance.

This theme is not the dilemma of art and of other aesthetic experiences. For I do not presume that the situation I have indicated is of importance only for the imaginative who may be more aware of it. We are but at the beginning of the cheating or, rather, recheating of whole-objects: the residues of an ancient environment, very largely destroyed already in the youth of us who are older, linger a little.

The fact is, again, that an uniformly robust awareness of whole-objects as such has always been rare, always hard-won. For neither has an environment of raw Nature, where practical life is restricted to a few simple operations, confirmed that awareness; a Nature all-powerful in every respect, whose dictates and whose look cannot be modified. This absence of scale or limit suggests for itself and tends to elicit from man omnipotence or other inordinate familiarity, often paranoid, a relationship with an invading-invaded object that at no time has been dissociated from individual and group projections. Attempted symbiosis with Nature in primitive societies discovers harmony by means of animism, of rites, of tabus, and even by means of the disfiguration of bodies to which I have referred. A specialized form of such partial and therefore absorbent relationship with objects is mysticism. Naturally we do not know whether the future promises a great extension of exotic religions. In an environment strictly ruled by technology, manic states produced by drugs will probably dispense with complicated faiths: except about the immediate needs of men there may be little stimulus to argument as far as cosmology is concerned. Therein lies a hope. On the other hand, just as it was inconceivable to an Australian native that the searching interior of that vast continent could be of a limited character, so the environment created by technological advance appears omnipotent. Already there is no way— worse—there is no reason in the light of which to modify or arrest. Practical benefits have been overwhelming.

But every perky car mascot has a whole-object under its belt.

NOTES

1. A. Stokes. *The Invitation in Art*. With a preface by Richard Wollheim (London, Tavistock Publications, 1965).
2. Lawrence Nield. *Architectural Forms originating in the House* (Lecture in Cambridge University School of Architecture, Easter Term, 1965).
3. *New Statesman*, 4 March 1966. *The Gutenberg Galaxy* (London, Routledge, 1962).

II. Michelangelo's *Giorno*

In the last chapter I have given reason for thinking that the future role of art will be even more important provided that culture continues as strongly to need vivifying symbols of whole-objects. We cannot be certain of continuation and it is not too soon to prepare ground for a struggle. We are in excellent position for corporate aesthetic resistance, for closure of ranks scattered throughout contemporary art, following the great dissemination of knowledge of art and of its understanding that modern methods of communication have caused. I believe that the first sign of that readiness must be the reinforcement of links that connect diverse manifestations of our contemporary art not only with the art of Oceanic or Cycladic culture, for instance, but with Western European art since the Renaissance; at the point, that is, where rupture has been celebrated and thereupon presumed; with the art of the past that we know best, the one perhaps the most varied and prolific and ambitious, the art of the societies that have gradually evolved our own.

The connection between our past and modern art that occupies this book is solely of a general kind. It embraces a theme common to all art, but in Europe the assertion of it has been the most daring or challenging whether we consider Michelangelo or collage, with which the next chapter is concerned.

To us the representation of correct musculature, however detailed, is no longer emotive in itself: we no longer associate naturalism *tout court* with the promise of aesthetic value. It has become more interesting, therefore, to ask why the spectator may be intensely moved in Michelangelo's Medici Chapel, San Lorenzo, by the musculature of the elbow of *Giorno's* twisted-back left arm and by the extraordinary bulges of the flattened hand. The spectator has the sensation not only of seeing clearly but of having thereby unravelled a complicated physiological structure that for most of us, even with the help of a photograph of an arm in this position, would seem vague and therefore unremarkable. It is moving and pleasurable to feel that we may possess in such a vivid detail the essence of Michelangelo's creativeness, an impression that would survive, I believe, if the detail were isolated from the figure and if we had no other experience of Michelangelo's sculpture. For there are rhythm and density that articulate for us, as well as the physique, the mind imputed to the figure or to its fragment: these are together not only a single but a crowded unit in our eyes.

Further, there is another and equally powerful concatenation of breathtaking virtuosity related to the first. To see it we must contemplate the whole marble block.

We are very conscious that as well as a piece of enlarged and powerful verisimilitude *Giorno* is undisguisedly an emaciated stone, partly rough. When viewed from the back the reclining, mountainous figure with long unsupported feet suggests the squat penury of a pebble. The reconciliations of the unsettled pose, an outcome of naturalistic aim at its most ambitious—and what was most ambitious technically tended at that moment of art to be most expressive also—are themselves subject to another astounding equilibrium between the extreme articulation of much of the figure and areas that have been, or partially have been, left as roughly chiselled stone. The restless Olympian *Giorno* emerges from the substance of the mountain with which the mattress of his hair and his roughed-out bearded face and angry eyes are cognate. All four *Times of the Day* are shrunken blocks: seen from the front the wide blunt knob of *Giorno's* head ruminates beyond

14

a deep crater and beyond the ridged right arm like peaks of the Carrara range that have been reduced by ancient quarrying, the scene for Michelangelo of many arduous months.

As a mountain may appear to transmit to itself the presence of its peak, so *Giorno's* square head, sunk in the shoulders, impregnates with thought and feeling the body's bulk: as if the brain were entirely a transmitter rather than the receiver also of corporeal sensations. *Our* sensation is that muscle speaks; there is speech not from the mouth but from contours and bulges that ripple at the behest of a reckless verisimilitude.

Now such communication more commonly proceeds from figurations that are greatly modified or generalized forms of physiological intricacy. Those partial abstractions have a closer correspondence with the visual residues left in the mind's eye when we contemplate our own feelings. That the unquiet real marble body, so to say, can have been made to reflect, to enlarge, this inner life becomes a triumph, not only for Michelangelo but for everyone: we are exalted.

We look to things for confirmation of cohesiveness and power. Here before us is a marble body not rarefied by the spirit but exhibiting the spirit, the inner life, first as a concrete, but then triumphantly as a naturalistic, form. Such grandeur of the intricate body, companion to the mountain, is dear to us. Indeed, nothing else in art offers as multiform a reassurance in spite of the huge melancholy inherent in the Medici sculptures.

It is considerable satisfaction when we feel in sculpture of the human body that the inwardly-conceived cylinder, let us say, an image-residue of contemplated mental states, has been translated into the outward terms of thigh and arm. Many experiences are brought to bear on any projection of the body that we judge to be somewhat comprehensive in this respect. And we often find in primitive or conventionalized art that a geometry of the inner life pervades an astonishing likeness to the outward model achieved by simplification, in terms of

15

an essence distilled. But the developed Antique, much of the Renaissance and pre-eminently Michelangelo have dispensed with essences, with those startling abstractions that encircle a particular likeness, in favour of conceptions of naturalistic truth infused with more grandiose abstractions borrowed from architecture and, in the case of Michelangelo, from a mountainous mineral strength as well. Instead of an adjusted cylinder for arm or leg we experience the elucidation of an anatomical network that refers fiercely to the inner life as do conventionalized schemata more slowly: we imagine an inner configuration to have now become no less palpable than a most intricate body and its daylight. Also we discover that between the rough mountain and ourselves there is the bridge of the countless stones broken and organized in a humanist architecture. Apprehending the sculpture's connection with mountain and with architecture, we embrace more material, more of the outside world, within the corporeal ambit of art. I shall suggest later that so extensive a corporeal realm corresponds both with the general compulsions of phantasy, and specifically with a main aesthetic component that results from what I shall again call 'carving' activity or conception.

These are connections which, when we view the Antique, may often appear dormant: they are instantly aroused by the low relief of the early Quattrocento and at the behest of Michelangelo. The period between the Antique and the Renaissance plays a very important part: we have in mind not only Giotto and Giovanni Pisano but huge monuments such as Pisa cathedral where the captive marbles of which they are made seem to affirm union not only with religion but even more with man's demand to see himself in their arched progressive tiers. The bias of the Antique and of the Renaissance towards verisimilitude is to be understood or appreciated only when beheld in harness with this intense feeling of ideal communion with ordered stone. The great innovator in painting, Masaccio, is inconceivable without that awareness.

Carved mineral mass was felt potentially to correspond with the *varied* riches of a monolithic self, to inspire in graphic art and sculpture a reconstruction of psyche by means of the complicated terms of anatomical animation. The material of art itself was for art corporeal substance. The originators in chief on the visual side of the first Italian Renaissance period were architects and carvers. There is emblematic justice in an old conception of fixing the inauguration of Renaissance art by the date 1402 or 1403 when Brunelleschi and the young Donatello are reputed to have paid together their first visit to Rome, that is, to the Roman ruins and sculpture.

The verisimilitude, the perspective, developed at that time, was a liberation from less vivid conventions whereby to project this birth of the freedom-loving body from the mother stones of architecture. Figures boldly emerge. The representation of movement was of its essence not only for this reason but because a turning body allowed of a more complicated and dramatic articulation. The twists of *Giorno's* arms, torso, and legs upon the inclined plane of the sarcophagus would emphasize a position of extreme discomfort were it not for the superabundant impression of power and control. Another art, not unrelated with European naturalistic sculpture, the classical ballet, similarly displays the body in open poses that do not excite a sense of strain but yet are, however static, never of a temper that is relaxed. It cannot be said that sculpture which followed Michelangelo, a giant of restlessness, conveys, as should ballet, an absence of strain. Yet if in the Medici chapel there is agony, or at least a top-heavy melancholy, there appear even so an overriding density and calm as well. One is reminded a little of both roots of this art, of Masaccio, who in the Brancacci chapel combined what were to be the two great themes of fifteenth-century painting; movement, chiaroscuro, stress, with an emphasis upon spatial interval, upon what was soon to become Pieroesque

17

calm. No accomplishment in painting is as comprehensive as Masaccio's. So often in art the greatest moments are the first.

It is dismaying, it appears mean and puritanical that some of our experts should still be antipathetic, as a matter of principle, to Florentine achievement in cases where they are so conscious of the striving towards naturalism upon which the attainment partly depended. Other aims in art have been less vulgarized without a doubt. But the fearsome aesthetic person is perfidious who rejects on principle the non-decorative fulsomeness of the early naturalism. He is rejecting a basis of art where it has been shown ambitiously, with many more aspects if also diffusely (except at supreme moments), the identification of inner organization of the spirit with the wholeness and articulation of the nude, and the identification of this image itself with the actuality of the substance or materials, especially meaningful in the case of carving, from which it is made or imaginatively derived.

III. Collages

Spectacular and even panoramic figuration, especially in the close-up, has now gained unlimited scope of a kind by means of the cinema, by means of photography.

The stricture that ends the last chapter does not embrace a plea for naturalistic art here and now. It refers to the connection that in my view is untouched—surely it could not be otherwise; it is hurtful to the understanding of art to deny it—between advanced illusionist techniques that used to thrive and their partial abandonment in the present. The qualification, 'partial', comes about because a total abandonment in painting is impossible. Wherever a two-dimensional area, wherever a surface suggests even a most shallow depth, the fabrication of visual illusion occurs. Indeed this tends to happen if any mark is made upon it [1].

In the developments I am about to discuss there is, however, entire abandonment of the studied imitation on a painted surface of objects in the outside world. What, then, is the crux of this revolt? I believe it centres on the fact that imitativeness, in that it involves the magnification of illusory effects, can be thought to separate the work of art from actuality and even from the actuality of the objects represented. But this has become obnoxious because illusion itself, in the form at any rate of phantasy, is regarded as necessitous or actual equally with the actuality of outside objects. Their wonderful mingling in naturalistic art was an imaginative creation no longer apposite to their alternation as we now experience it without much help, and without a present possibility of desiring the help, from reductive cultural filters. I hope to make this clearer.

Professor Isaiah Berlin pointed out in one of his lectures on *Some Sources of Romanticism* that just before the turn of the nineteenth century, Tieck asked the actors for an interruption that destroyed the dramatic illusion in a play he wrote. The actors would then talk together in a matter-of-fact or cynical manner that rejected the play as such. Isaiah Berlin pointed out that this qualifying of make-believe by actuality to the extent that they were interchanged, achieved a full expression over a hundred years later at the time of Dada [2].

The reaction against unrelieved make-believe persists. Neither real objects nor the phantasies they stimulate are now felt necessarily to be as uniformly pliable as their transformation into the ingredients that furnish a make-believe. The simplicity of this amalgam has undergone many attacks, many vicissitudes, in the last eighty years. Actuality and phantasy can be regarded as partners, and equal partners at that. Reduce actuality, and you are reducing the character of phantasy as such. Phantasy, projections, symbolic constructions, are no longer considered gratuitous, 'unreal', even imaginative. They reflect psychic structure and hence form the root of art. Phantasy and actuality do not only curb each other: 'straight' actuality is in fact the origin of 'straight' phantasy. Thus the modern sculptor does not begin to disguise the stone that he works. There is the stone and there is the stone that is made evocative, an incipient dualism of factors that more usually have been in varying degrees in closer amalgam, for the comprehensive culture of the fifteenth century especially, and for the subsequent art of Michelangelo.

It was in fact poets who first of our time employed a bared dualism. Since many words have numerous overtones, it became important to allow to them their varied actuality even while they were pressed into the service of a narrow theme; a consideration that has led to an employment of images forged from juxtaposed, previously dissociated parts, of metaphor divorced from simile, an interplay of matter-of-factness with a poetic intent. Much fragmentation—Dadaist inversions even—attributable to avant-garde art in many media is due to some loosening of the ancient cultural amalgam that in make-believe compounds figuration with everyday, contradictory experience and with actual substances.

Art for a century has often assumed a form that the past would have considered practice dress: in the highly theatrical presentations of the conventional ballet it is this that of recent years has sometimes been the costume.

For a long time now painters of *all* reputable schools have had no interest in disguising the flatness or actuality of the picture plane for the sake of *trompe l'oeil* alone; or in concealing the process by which art is made: an undisguised and even exaggerated process has become a prime instrument of aesthetic value. We have had poems that for many readings remain little more than words and music that to an unsympathetic hearing is literally only sounds, only disjointed, far-separated noises even; but it is obvious that visual art, commanding sight and touch, is strongest in the presentation of actuality, with far the widest range.

As the sole framework for European painting massive illusionism was bound up with biblical and historical recreation; with the rendering of stabilizing myths and beliefs that could appear to encompass actuality. None of this would now possess a cultural incisiveness and a reference also to the psychic actuality of the inner life: in sum, such representations, though they were made for us with distinction, would not serve with urgency as symbols of whole and self-sufficient objects. An arrant, personal employment of symbolism by many artists, very notably by Picasso in *Guernica*, may appear to mitigate that situation. Not even Picasso can help to stabilize a culture that lacks a systematic and deeply-founded symbolism. He, as much as anyone, has shown us that as a result of the protesting Romantic Movement, culture no

21

longer controls a symbolic language of comprehensive use.

Today, instead of the steady arms of culture we have juxtaposition, in the first place the juxtaposition, often in preference to the mingling, of actuality and phantasy. Moreover the confusing juxtapositions inherent in our experience of the technological environment have to be stated, if only because they cannot be fully comprehended or interpreted. Surrealist art, of course, is contrived out of unexpected juxtapositions. Often, it seems, they misfire. It is of particular interest that any such condemnation has not always been considered of the first importance, at least theoretically. An emptiness, a destruction, has been exhibited as such. So called anti-art has had an important place in pioneering. A chance conglomeration might amplify the ceaseless meaningless shocks from the juxtapositions to which urban life is subject. That the shock of juxtaposition—the juxtaposition even of destruction or evanescence with construction—in contemporary art has become a requirement prior even to the often very evident poetry desired and discovered in the process, is perhaps illustrated by the fact that the power of an antiquated *trompe-l'oeil* imitativeness has served as an avant-garde method in Surrealist hands when used to transmit the shock of unexpected conjunctions.

The brassy element of shock, impact, or arrest has of course always been present in art. Craft to the ends of verisimilitude partakes of this surprise quality that is often the necessary preliminary, the very form, of the invitation to join and merge with the presentation. It is significant that even the academic art of the day tends to disrupt any value it might transmit by the imposition of grating vulgarity or crudity. What has gone, what cannot be recaptured, is a cultural or subsuming style, native to the art of more integrated, less questioning societies, by which to arrest, to invite, and to figure forth. And whereas the creation of art has always depended upon a successful bringing together of the divergent, upon unifying effects that contrast, we must now make art out of confronting elements that tend to evoke for themselves, it seems, a cultural principle that only in an obscure, non-masterful sense can be said to have been imposed. A sign of this humility or partial capitulation, certainly of the dominating experimental verve, lies in the process of making a collage compared with the process of painting. A new piece added to a collage may most forcibly re-direct the structural and emotional conception to a degree that could not have been anticipated [3]. There are compensations in the strong impact and often in the purity of composition released from a variety of trammels, particularly subject matter; in the employment of actual, formed objects or of an unexpected weighty substance as implements of the urgent spirit however vague its voice. The actuality of heavy sanded surfaces created by Dubuffet and Tapies brings their work of this kind close to collage. On the other hand some artists, as I have mentioned, seek to make capital out of the fugitive propensities of matter, to harness decay or destruction to the purposes of art, a pile of distorted mineral rubbish. All these faceless insistent products crowd in upon us as if we were blind. Pygmalion's model now carries off a far more vivid dash than does he. We are up against the modern artifact as if our own paler history were composed of confrontations that produced their dominant overtones as a result of a similar transposition of the context. Indeed, that is a fair generalization about the development of psychic structure.

At the same time the employment in collages and assemblages of actual objects points not only to the reiteration of whole-object nature in a void created by the abandonment of representations that truly imitate them, but also to our particular hunger in modern environment for surrounding objects that we may contemplate in their possession of the wholeness and self-sufficiency of which the nude was once the

23

presiding symbol. For it will be said in the last chapter that our attitudes to actuality as such, at any rate to the concrete media of the arts, project a continuous reference to a rudimentary body that corresponds with the corporeal content of phantasy in general; the more so where the actuality of the medium is stressed.

Blindly, like the infant with his part-objects, we grope for those attributes as this art pounds us. We have come to conceive from such works that they possess a significance in their quality of bright or insistent objects prior to their particular value of which that fresh impact could be the proof. Hence in general their great if often unfocussed power over us; and it is to the impact, it seems to me, rather than to the ordering of the cosmos, that we attend in looking at a Mondrian or at constructivist art in any form or, indeed, at the first great Cubist art; though, naturally, there follows the significance that is in line with the artist's aim without which a meaningful object could not have been created.

'When, as in a primitive cult object, a shell becomes a human eye because of its context, the accepted hierarchy of categories becomes disrupted' [4]: the confrontation wrought by a changed context. This principle of collage and assemblage is by no means new; not the principle. What of the scarecrow, of Valentines, Ex-votos, intarsia, gold keys and haloes in Gothic paintings? What of mosaic? The question could be made very long. A confrontation and a degree of correspondence have always been sought, by sculptors particularly, between physical material and the complication, aggregation, and resolving of mental states which may be suggested particularly by natural objects in a new and varied context. The thread of this activity has not only not been broken but has been strengthened by modern artists. I have tried to show that naturalism, a varying degree of illusionism (though in truth very rarely its most complete expressions) could manipulate this thread no less than other styles; but in so far as naturalism of all kinds has now gone by the board, painting approximates more literally either to sculpture or to architecture, to the arts in which the materials themselves have always manifestly retained their own significance whatever their transposition to a new context. Not, I repeat, that naturalistic painting was without what I have long called 'carving' values, that is to say the values in which especially colour and disposition of space play the part (in combination with other parts) that can be summed by the expression 'enlivenment of the surface', an activity in contrast with, no less than in combination with, what I have called modelling activity that creates the looming of forms, rhythm, movement, stress, and strain. In actual carving the intrusive chisel enlivens the stone, a material of unrestrained imaginative value unlike the clay, a more homogeneous substance of which nothing is expected in art except a pliability, a wholesale lending of itself, for the fashioning of the artist's imagery. I have often suggested that with the breakdown of deeply meaningful stone or brick architecture in the middle of the last century, the role of providing satisfying surfaces was first taken over by painters: it is shown by the increased interest of the paint's textures as if that tinted mud were a vivifying agent of canvas or board. Collage has enlivened the picture plane with salvaged pieces of our staccato environment adapted to the role of a prolixity upon this plane.

A substance to be carved, I must repeat, unlike the moulded clay, is a potential ready-made, an object fit to be contemplated in isolation, to some degree an *objet trouvé* an overriding sense of whose actuality usually persists whatever the sculptor does with it. It may be the grain of stone or wood of which we are so persistently conscious, the texture, and it can be the marble landscape or mountain when the hand is Michelangelo's. We are at times even more aware of that combination in great stone architecture where forms and

25

adamantinem aterial connive. The arts of collage and assemblage, it is easy to see, are not of a different genus though the pieces of the external world are taken from their usual context and stuck together not in order to create, it is true, an illusion of some other natural object nor a shelter, but a meaning transmitted by physical objects as such that in their combination is wider than their own. Hence the often abrupt evocative encounters of differing flotsam, imitative or reflective of emotional collocations among the accidents and contradictions to which environment subjects us, the fleeting amalgam that this art both satirizes and attempts to pin down, to make poetic, whole. So great has been the influence of collage that much painting now combines with sculpture, or at least with materials used in a relief that bear witness to a predominance of 'carving' values as has been said, though the reliefs are usually made by impositions. There is a similar connection with collage in the work today of many pure sculptors. I see in this context the generous steel constructions of David Smith. His delicately abraded piled cubes provide a countenance for steel and for welded construction, but not at all an expressionist countenance for robots. His is a deeply satisfying achievement that enlivens our sense of a substance forced on us today, making for its use a connection with the anthropomorphic carving of stone and even more widely with man's vivification of the landscape through several thousand years, particularly with his cutting of the trays of mounting terraces. Out of fire and shrill piercing, out of sharp usage, an anatomy has been forged of great breadth for metal.

This liberty to serve materials as such has hitherto been rare in the arts outside those that are professedly assistant or decorative; whereas today the independence allowed to actuality, to materials, immanent in what I have called the 'carving' principle which magnifies interpenetration with an expressiveness beyond them, is the root of much excellence in our art. For it is no time not to use stuff as such, no time to sublimate material, disguise the medium or even to have a medium in so far as this word implies its utter subjection. Submission to some extent to the medium is a method by which the artist seeks to construct a home for us in an environment that is as yet far from being a confident projection of the body with its eyes that we can see. It is as if we were blind and as if what hits us so hard is blind also. New art is not out of step with the old though the gap be wide between our faceless art of material and the lengthy bodies that the paintings in the National Gallery have imposed on existence.

We sometimes mistake a collage for a painting, and we find that our feelings about the object alter materially when the truth is known. I become aware in that situation of closure as if a writing on the wall has itself been walled up. The entire collage that successfully counterfeits a painting tends, when we know, to diminish our sense of a transmission between artist and spectator. The material has won over the artist: the work has now become at one remove like a print, though in the case of many prints the handiwork is no less evident than in front of a painting. But in the case of collage we are aware also of a craft that is self-concealing, of a fitting together that we associate with furniture-making rather than with an expressive use of paint. Even Matisse's cut-outs, though they show his subtle manipulation of the scissors, do not convey to us the continuity in organizing *matière* for which we look in his painting: a comparable conspiracy with the canvas has not occurred; indeed the background is not canvas but paper, the same material as the gummed papers. It will seem arbitrary, therefore, that I have associated collage so strictly with the 'carving' aspect of visual art. Moreover collage is always superimposition like one piece of clay worked into another. On the other hand it is not difficult to see that Schwitters's collages cause waste material, as well as the surface on which it adheres, to be precious. He elicited gems: it is as if not the stone but the dull ungleaming clay had

27

been made to irradiate. In carving, no part of the material should serve only as a foil to other parts: the gems transmute the character, exalt the potentiality, of the setting. Carving tends to moderate the overriding gesture to which the clay easily lends itself. Intrusive though it be, perhaps in compensation, the act of carving tends to favour gradual forms, a wider spreading of accents and emphases: the material, like space in a painting by Piero della Francesca is uniformly valued, just as each of his colours is uniformly valued, that is to say not considered dominant, nor subject to, but brotherly with, the other colours. In an earlier book I have associated this aspect of visual art more closely with the re-creation of self-sufficient or whole objects in distinction from the incantatory power of modelling, a partner that extends our grasp of objects and thus reinforces and inspires part-object relationship. In my view, then, in spite of the superimposition entailed, the art of collage and the influence of collage upon painting and upon sculpture have strengthened the 'carving' approach to visual art, the sense of the independent object, the actuality of the material whose actuality, we shall see, symbolizes both the body and naked mental structures.

The Cubist art of Braque and Picasso wherein collage first appeared, can now be reckoned as the most intense and most varied 'carving' attainment of modern art. Those artists' introduction of *papier collé*, of more substantial objects also, were means—never forgotten since—that they invented to increase object-nature partly in the place of direct imitation. Thereafter substances, objects, stranger to each other than the announcements with emendatory diagonal strips on advertisement boards, insist on the assimilation of rival gestures and new contexts.

The intrusive character of collage—we have seen that this too connects with carving—has been exploited far more widely than the efflorescence of surfaces which appeals to me more. The latter has influenced the painters who sparsely stain canvases of the finest grain, whereas the former aspect has influenced painters—Picasso at one time among them—who intrude a flat shape that at first sight seems foreign to the rest [5]: so imported does that part of the surface appear that we approach in perplexity to discover whether collage has in fact been used.

A combination of an impersonal element with expressiveness, collage has become the most distinctive invention of modern art. Nauseated by the bill-board—one of the progenitors, to be sure, of collage as of pop art so much later—we continue to find solace in a beautiful mosaic of paper scraps or in *collage déchiré*. An impersonal weathered surface is precious to us, a record of our past that cannot signal through a precise semaphore, a residue of the life from within that once informed as secretly the stones of well-worn towns.

In the first chapter I have hinted that for modern urban life our eyes and other senses no longer receive nor as easily construct the broader symbolic impressions of whole-objects in terms of that environment: there appears to the contemplative mind a drag upon many individual things as such, a partial dissolution of a self-sufficiency that depends from the imaginative angle upon the notion of a wide organization, as well as upon the frequency, of valued things. Modern art shows that we must search for mere fragments of an organization and that we have an entire impatience with cultural symbolic systems: they would lack impetus. They cannot be applied now to the order or, rather, to the lack of order, of things.

It is certain that in the figurative sphere no artist has rivalled Giacometti's hunt for an intrinsic residue among his life-long companions of what in other times might amply have been the stranger; the stranger with the meaning attributed to him on the first pages; a symbolic whole-object briefly encountered, a unit within a self-supporting *mise-en-scène*. Much

visual art today has abandoned this direct search for an unconquerable quiddity of the self, an occupation of Romantic
thinking right through to the Existentialist version of the
present time, in favour of the sifting for the parallel term, for
the unconquerable natural or manufactured object, the ordinary objects of the outside world stripped or cleaned of our
easier modes of appropriation by projection and of their
subservience from the imaginative point of view to facile
emotions and memories. These are now held to be lying side
by side with the objects that stimulate them, a small but meaningful separation. One aspect of Alain Robbe-Grillet's novels
illustrates it. Things are; they are out there: as seen with the
eye of an artist they are meticulously described again and
again for their cursory form at the cost of dramatic progression. From time to time we experience in reading Robbe-
Grillet the wonder we would feel if actors on the stage were
to say nothing, were to abandon acting as in the Tieck drama,
an ideal situation to which several of Beckett's presentations
approximate.

And so there is now a code of aesthetic reverence for the
mere presence of things, for a residual presence in whatever
way this may be formulated. Such formulation, of course,
betrays more than an element of projection: it makes meaningful, as always in art, a new appraisement implied for the
opposite arm, for inner or psychic structure difficult to seize
and little known. Hence an impatience with all myths enveloping the physical world, a disquiet not over the sublimation
of this or that tendency but over the cultural veils by which
sublimation has dulled the ache for psychic actuality, for
psychic truth as far as repression allows us to entertain it.
Self-knowledge has been obstructed not only by ourselves
but by the wholesale interpretation of behaviour and of objects presented by all societies. We feel it to be so today only
because we have science together with a culturally bare world.
Once, every form of knowledge and understanding tended to

coalesce. They are more likely today to be disparate. The findings of psycho-analysis have been very little accepted beyond their generality; yet the rejected rumour of them has been enough to curb, to eliminate even, much systematic rationalization of omnipotence.

Some painters explore relationships to objects so manifold that the attempt is sometimes made *not* to conceive the work of art as a closed system, closed against the contingent circumstances of its viewing [6]. Will art press on to join all the accidents of nature and, through an excess of the 'carving' principle, expire?

Meanwhile there is considerable pathos, there is even an element of drama, in any comfort gained from an imaginative permissiveness that extends to objects an opaque identity that has eluded our possessiveness. Objects have become mysterious; we are sometimes unable to establish a progressive visual system from part- to whole-objects. Not only the urban environment but even technological exploration projected on to paper tends to blur divergence between them. I instanced the magnified form of the artist's thumb, a reversal of scale that seems to tally with our new universe though a part of the human body is not usually in question. Indecision multiplies; it was the artist's aim to transfer that indecision to his thumb since the enlargement of objects by magnifying aids, particularly by photography, has forced on us startling units of organization not apparent to the unreinforced senses. The result in much pictorial art has been the exploitation of the disruption of scale, and the great modern invention of sparse design on a huge canvas (with or without a sea of paint). Totally ambiguous in scale, these works may appear to expand further, to grow over us, very complete though they be in themselves as well. In this way an extreme part-object possessiveness returns. Tobey's minute working also cannot be kept at a distance: we don't know whether his marks approximate to big things made small or

31

to things smaller than his forms made big [7]: without figuration or without an architectural format, an architectural context, this ambiguity becomes likely in regard to scale, and consequently the overreaching effect that is much valued. It has stemmed in the first place from the intimate quality of naïve or primitive art wherein the attempt is made to mirror the artist's active as well as contemplative involvement with objects for which, whether they be animal or mineral, he discovers a manner of communal arrest that brings them closer into our possession. Scale is sometimes reversed in this art. It is absent again in the equivocal yet blinding chromatic researches of Op art: it is absent in aesthetic products that have in large part been derived from engineering and mathematical elisions: these works can entail also a perplexing reference to an inner world that the wary artist seems to have circumvented: they may even brandish a simplicity that appears to have no bond either with ourselves or with object-nature as formerly envisaged.

But though we are unable to establish objects in an ordered hierarchy that satisfies the imagination, most artists still proclaim that objects are 'there', that the world 'is'; that any amplification might qualify, might confuse, the impression of 'is-ness'. I believe this attitude could be interpreted as follows: the faith persists that the good inner object, the core of the ego, survives (cf p. 8); but it is unlikely to dominate. This good object has insufficient power to integrate with itself all the other psychic factors in so far as we tend to destroy the integrity, as we conceive it, of objects through excessive projective identification and other schizoid mechanisms that eventually bring about chaos in the inner world.

The manner of our art betrays a mixed condition; it is, of course, over-determined. I do not go back on what I wrote about 'is-ness' in *Three Essays on the Painting of our Time* [8]. Thus as well as some humility before objects, some idolatry of the actual, an old omnipotence may be exploiting a manic and predominantly dismissive rule especially over those artistic happenings wherein the only figure is the wilful engineering of chance effects at the expense of selection, at the expense of scale.

But I think there is a sense also in which the abandonment of imitation for the use of actual things in collages and assemblages partakes of a stubborn, unidealized affirmation that the good objects, whole and part, survive, if barely; exist, if fitfully. From that beginning—pious hopes are cheap—we may in art eventually proceed to construct more generally whole-objects that are rich; to re-construct the nude; to revise in the name of psychic truth a sober conception of the integrated being.

NOTES

1. RICHARD WOLLHEIM. *On Drawing an Object* (London, H. K. Lewis, 1965). I place much reliance on this finding.
2. BBC THIRD PROGRAMME August-September 1966. A recording of the lectures given under the auspices of the Bollingen Foundation at the National Gallery of Art, Washington, in April 1965.
3. ANDREW FORGE in conversation with the author, who owes to Forge the suggestion that he should write about collage.
4. WILLIAM C. SEITZ. *The Art of Assemblage* (New York, Museum of Modern Art, 1961).
5. ROBERT MELVILLE in conversation with the author.
6. ANDREW FORGE. *Rauschenberg* (New York, Harold Abrams, 1967).
7. LIONEL BURMAN. 'The Paradox of Scale' (*The British Journal of Aesthetics*, Vol. 6, No. 4, October 1966).
8. London, Tavistock Publications, 1961.

IV. Art and Embodiment

The biological aims of the instincts that drive us are often imagined to possess some other meaning. Yet the processes of thought at the service of instinct (even when led to think otherwise) do not dispose any explanation of living and dying beyond the terms of instinctual necessity. The deeper purpose of living is but the common factor in all the contingent purposes, and truth about dying is the dying.

It may be best to enter into some harmony with that conclusion: a momentary acceptance comes by brooding on the fact that many valued states of being are self-sufficient. Those that are contemplative sublimate instinctual drive and yet in some degree they mirror the narrowness of instinctual purposiveness since these states are valued as ends-in-themselves even though their merit has a considerable repercussion on our lives. Our enjoyment of aesthetic value entails contemplative acts which can be held to reconcile us somewhat to the narrowness of biological necessity: they are emotional and intellectual exercises largely innocent of teleological tautology.

But contemplation of such 'useless' objects is not alone in possessing so wise a value. Even team games can sometimes show that there is a premium in ritual though it be shorn of its occasion: the game has become intensified as a spectacle though outdistancing the express purpose of a contest: the value is now wholly in a wider symbolic happening, in following the rules, in being subject to the climate and to other forms of chance and 'natural selection'. So withdrawn an event is often refreshing; and the appreciation of art is particularly so whenever the self-sufficiency of other experiences has been at the greatest discount.

But of course it is impossible to reserve the value of contemplative states only to their correction of unbridled teleological attitudes that are themselves in large part necessary to living. We can sufficiently re-arrange the picture if we think for a moment of the projections that will be induced during the contemplation of a natural scene, as we look at leafy laden trees, for instance, that appear retreated into happiness: they hold for us our belief in goodness and love by which we live: we personalize thereby attachment to objects. The attempt to explore the good beyond its first objectives, beyond its first necessity for the continuance of living, reflects the number of enemies to which the good is exposed. On the other hand the contemplative state denotes as well a power of potential detachment, of a detachment not from life but from some of the compulsions to simplify the forceful yet ambiguous stream. Contemplation, it appears to me, indeed consciousness itself, implies the potential attainment of a degree of acceptance, of a viewing that divides us from some concern at least, doubtless in the interest of the death to which we are no less subject than to the compulsion of sustaining and improving life. Some total acceptance will also be implicit in the apprehension of those happy trees [1].

Contemplation implies reference to the forms of the outside world: even the self as the contemplated object requires the recall of sensations: in art there is no attempt whatsoever to separate the person from his body: the body is so primary an object that a sense of it will not be absent from the relationships to any other object. All the detail of this obvious admission—it is the detail, of course, that provides force—will have been derived from the researches of psycho-analysis. If we try to contemplate the psycho-analytic literature as a whole, we might conclude that the extent of reasonableness and emotional stability in our attitudes *vis-à-vis* objects, human, animal, vegetable, and mineral, depends in the first place on the degree to which, under the stress of frustration, conflict, fixation, trauma, and so on, we have integrated our love, hate, and envy of bodily function, the degree to which thoughts about one zone of the body have not been confused with thoughts about another zone [2], the degree to which all functions are *felt* in the recesses of the mind as parts of a single and varied entity.

The balanced emotional estimation of the body is an ideal. One may doubt whether any human being has attained entire integration of those hidden feelings. It remains the quest, an impetus of adult search including the one of art. Indeed the contribution of art is quickly apparent; for instance in regard to the huge concern particularly of the infant and the child—a concern, therefore, that will always considerably persist—about the inside of the body, though the nearest even to an intuitive formulation at which most people arrive is in the context of hypochondria and psychosomatic illness when these conditions have been recognized for what they are.

Whereas the art of the written word is with difficulty and indirectness centred on this matter, portraits and paintings of the figure are less hard to interpret. Rembrandt, it seems to me, painted the female nude as the sagging repository of jewels and dirt, of fabulous babies and magical faeces despoiled yet later repaired and restored, a body often flaccid and creased yet still the desirable source of a scarred bounty: not the bounty of the perfected, stable breast housed in the temple of the integrated psyche that we possess in the rounded forms of classical art, but riches and drabness joined by the infant's interfering envy, sometimes with the character of an oppressive weight or listlessness left by his thefts. There supervenes, none the less, a noble acceptance of ambivalence in which love shines.

This is not necessarily to hint at Rembrandt's emotional equipment nor to stigmatize a bias in seventeenth-century northern European culture. On the contrary the contrasting classical conception is very rare: it is far more common to discover in art the implication with the inside of the body: we accept it that the Athenian achievement is without parallel and that the emptiness and falsity to which the Greek ideal would often be reduced (though the inspiration will never disappear) could cause it to be less accessible even to some who, like Rembrandt, studied and borrowed from classical composition, learning especially how to achieve the look of inevitability whereby to dominate the larger aspects of design.

Rembrandt constructed a stable format out of contrary emotions, from a varied human condition to which he allowed by the granular additiveness of his technique, the progression to a munificence that crowns other impressions like a gratitude that has finally overcast an envy. He has shown in sum, as Kenneth Clark said of his portraiture, 'the raw material of grace' [3], strands of negative feeling, for instance, about the body limited to the original zones, a process that will have entailed some withdrawal of those parts of the self that have been sent into the object to plunder or to command; for otherwise the affirmation that I am I and they are they, an objective of art, cannot be clearly stated.

We are intact only in so far as our objects are intact. Art of whatever kind bears witness to intact objects even when the subject matter is disintegration. Whatever the form of transcript the original conservation or restoration is of the mother's body [4]. And whereas pictorial art employs and stimulates those infantine phantasies—they are many—that utilize the eyes for omnipotent projections, for omniscience, it enlarges upon the reassuring endurance of objects in the shadow of this attack: they are enthroned by the artist by means of a pictorial settlement wherein they may surrender themselves only to that multiform composition which symbolizes the integrated elements of the self no less than of the other person.

And yet almost every product of the body as well as disease, malformation, malfunction, and the inside itself (apart from ancient bone) continue to revolt us since we are implicated; not so much because we belong to a similar vulnerable organism but because attacking wishes have caused the imperfection of others to appear revengeful: that imperfection is likely to reflect also our own, split off in accordance with the necessities of narcissistic estimates. Every virtue resides or is symbolized in the flesh together with all humiliation, threat, and squalor. A moment of active grandeur may come with birth of the baby from inside; birth is sometimes a supreme event for the parents' reconciliation of phantasies about the body. Adult sexuality, adult love, can make every endowment commensurate. On the other hand an access of virtuosity for confusion and splitting may characterize this sphere. Success, full satisfaction, depends upon the disposition thereby involved of the early psychic structures regarding the body. As heretofore, not only do we project but we introject, including our own projections with their objects. Others, or parts of others, are inside us; parts of our bodies sometimes merit a double nomenclature: nor are these strangers likely to be at peace.

The medical view of the body is the most vivid and careworn of unemotional systems, a routine insistence that the body is a valuable machine. Concomitant with the growth and triumph of science there has occurred in culture a boastful surrender to the omnipresence of phantasy and finally in our own time a plain admission of compulsiveness. This, in my view, is the essence and origin of the Romantic Movement in the shadow of which we still live. The growth of science and the first rumbling of the Industrial Revolution killed the Enlightenment, the Age of Reason. As we have noted in the use to which actuality is put by the art of collage, actuality, and therefore the gaze of science, isolates and elicits phantasy as a stupendous force. A part of the aesthetic stress upon the actual is stress upon the corporeal content in phantasy.

We have learned that to examine how scored and pitted

smooth skin looks under the microscope does not help us to conceive the satin flesh as leather, to link conceptions of youth and age, to join our feelings about attractiveness and about repulsiveness in a form of truth or just accountancy. Yet even the handshake points to the expectation of a fundamental warmth, a requirement that never passes though it conflicts with a variety of contrary feelings about the person. Many have tried, therefore, when genital attraction is not notably involved, to value not the body but its animation, the life infusing the carcase that cannot in fact be separated from it. The once useful conception, the 'soul', is entirely outmoded in an age whose range of actualities continues to increase. We cannot dissociate people from their physical presence and we may sometimes fail to dissociate the presence that they present to us from the life of their persons under all circumstances. Narcissistic esteem, self-love, a fount of warm and generous estimates, does not confine its dealings to the soul. Love is as comprehensive as hate, though even within the narrow gauge that we are set by our compulsions there is much concerning which our feelings fluctuate. The intact objects, works of art, are a model for the direction of those feelings, not so much in reference to people specifically loved or hated but in the matter of the persons of our fellowmen more generally. A degree of education is possible and any profit from it may accrue to the intense relationships also. It is therefore important to discover in art the recounting of all aspects that the body has possessed, the inside (as seen from without) as well as the outside. (Thus the glimmering or tufted finery that clothes many sombre Rembrandt figures can mirror the character of *inner* objects for whose state the individual is massively responsible.)

It is for such communication, however recondite, that we scan good portraits. At any rate we learn to see the spirit, the animation, in terms of art's inoffensive material. That material stands for the body whether or not it has been used to represent the body. Art, truly seen, is never ghostly; and art, truly seen, does not so much educate us about animation, about the mind or spirit, about the intentions of others good or bad in which we find a source of persecutory feeling or of trust, as about the resulting body-person, about the embodiment that is much more than an embodiment because bodily attributes have always been identified with those intentions. A painting of the nude, therefore, is but one of the corporeal lessons set by art. There is a sense in which all art is of the body, particularly so in the eyes of those who accept that the painted surface and other media of art represent as a general form, which their employment particularizes, the actualities of the hidden psychic structure made up of evaluations and phantasies with corporeal content.

Though the emotion aroused may seem infinite, the variation of form is restricted: there is no merit in two heads or three legs. The forms that embrace what is most desirable and most rejected partake of an extreme limitation like the picture within its frame, like the meagre repertory of forms that are available to the artist. The grey haberdashery of an old man's loose flesh against a pillar of a swimming bath seems to negate the tie with the column's marble corporeality, while upon the stage in the second act of *The Sleeping Princess* the bodies of the radiant dancers transcend the paste-board palace and the very light. In both settings it is the architecture that provides both a mean and a continuo.

The thinking of art about the body is not hurried: the 'carved' medium and the animation are affirmed together as well as separately: the reaction-formation that divides the sensuous from the mental or spiritual is denounced. Art, and art alone, always haunted the position that of late psychoanalysis has fortified impregnably with deep-dug entrenchments; particularly modern art, at any rate in regard to an insistent respect paid to the prevalence of unorganized and

40

confusing phantasy that encircles actuality; the raw material to be organized.

I have stressed the whole-object nature to be envisaged when painting a nude. At the same time the artist attempts to formulate a coherence between the objects of which the self is partly composed and even to recall those parts that were split off and sent to live in other objects. We have seen in the context of collage and assemblage that contemporary art sometimes rejects imitation and employs an actual outside object brought into contact with other actual objects. Thereupon collage joins up with all art since it is ensemble, not the constituents, that constructs the whole-object we call a work of art. Behind the making and appreciation there is the hope of estimating human beings, at the very least the mere interaction of body and mind, in the way we contemplate and love artifacts, as well as in the light of other models.

The word 'contemplate' indicates at this point a state wherein further projective and splitting activities are at a discount in favour of the wider recognition of the object as a complete object. Nevertheless whatever aesthetic object we contemplate, it serves also as a symbol for an aspect, or for many aspects, of our accumulated feelings and projections and introjections in regard to the body to which in our own selves and in the case of others we are tied not only indissolubly but without a solution, without an integration continuous and stable; that is to say, incompletely when compared with a work of art *per se* whose medium is always broadly of its fabric. It is surely a modest and indispensable ideal that art proclaims.

A word finally about the great classical art of Western Europe that seems out-dated. It cannot be too strongly emphasized that at best this ideal treatment of the psyche and of the body has not involved denial and an averted gaze: it would otherwise be of no value. A perennial shapeliness in

41

classical art affirms a resolute hold upon the figure of the good breast installed in the psyche, enduring under the circumstances even of death and tragedy. Wherever the belief convinces, the tenacity corresponds with psychic truth in regard to the core of the strong ego and the fount of integration or successful development. To have been able to subsume under the aegis of so grand and active a manner in art a huge diversity of emotional experience has surely been among the greatest achievements of man.

There are many aspects: the alternative need not be between classical and anti-classical. In the *oeuvre*, for instance, of Matisse we witness an angular, pointed attack bent, even forced we may feel, into the round by his wry contentment with the enveloping rays of the sun. He contrived sumptuousness from colour so that the angular subsists as a simplicity in harmony with elegance. He reconciled the sumptuous with the meagre, the lavish and monumental with the thin, and the easy contentment of the decorative with what is stark, with an expressiveness that is circumscribed but not suppressed by the range of his opulence. That opulence would appear a surfeit were it not so neat an expression of the clinging to beneficence amid an angular and impatient world.

This lesson, the sharp lesson of Matisse who was neither classical nor expressionist, has not been overlooked by countless modern painters.

Art, we have seen in these pages, has always employed concrete, indeed corporeal, conceptions. The attempt has once more been made to exalt the truth and wisdom of art particularly in the light of its 'carving' component. The lesson that all art teaches rather than the survival of a living style is what matters first. But the present aesthetic submission to natural phenomena, even to chance confrontations, whereby art tends, closer than ever before, to embrace the process of nature—kinetic sculptures are physico-bodies that 'live' with us—might portend in the course of time a disappearance of art as we have understood it. This would matter not at all if a dilution of art proper were to mean that almost everyone has become an artist in the way of his work, in an area of his interests, in the manner that he views the world.

NOTES

1. A. STOKES. 'On Being Taken out of Oneself' (*Int. J. Psycho-Anal.* Vol. 47, Part 4, 1967).
2. DONALD MELTZER. *The Psycho-Analytical Process* (London, Heinemann, 1967).
3. KENNETH CLARK. *Rembrandt and the Italian Renaissance* (London, Murray, 1966).
4. There is particularly one detail among many that may help to indicate their scope, namely a psycho-analytic view of the mother's body not only as the target for the infant's first drives but also as a medium of communication and of defence against aspects of those drives in view of the mother's capacity to receive projections 'and to return to the infant parts of itself and its internal objects divested of all persecutory qualities by means of the feeding relation to the breast'. DONALD MELTZER, 'The Introjective Basis of Polymorphous Tendencies in Adult Sexuality' (*The British Psycho-Analytical Society and the Institute of Psycho-Analysis. Scientific Bulletin*, 1966, No. 7).

THE IMAGE IN FORM
A LECTURE

The Image in Form

Often in a talk [1] about art we get at least a partial division of formal attributes from representation. We say the formal relationships organize the representation, the images, on view. That's the traditional approach. On the other hand, in the theory of Significant Form, form is isolated from imagery, from the construction of likenesses in visual terms.

I am going to argue that formal relationships themselves entail a representation or imagery of their own though these likenesses are not as explicit as the images we obtain from what we call the subject matter. When later I shall refer to Cézanne's *Bathers* in the National Gallery, I shall suggest that there is far more imagery in this picture than the imagery of nudes in a landscape, a more generalized imagery, with references to all sorts of experiences, which proceeds from the formal treatment. Now I think one can say that that's obvious and indeed that it is presumed in the work of all the best writers today on current art; but it doesn't seem to have given rise to a really wide investigation of what is involved. I am going to make some suggestions about this.

The phrase 'the image in form' cropped up when I was asked to decide between two constructions at a Soto exhibition. They are made of projecting square plaques against a background of black and white lines. I said I thought one communicated a stronger image than the other. It suggested an image for an amalgam of experiences, even though that impression had not been achieved by the creation of a correspondence with recognized events as is the case where you have a subject matter. I found this abstract work to possess

47

an image all the same, whose character would not be alto-gether dissimilar in the long run for those who are able to lend themselves to abstract art.

Formal arrangements can sometimes transmit a durable image. That is not merely to say that they are expressive. There is a sense in which every object of the outside world is expressive since we tend to endow natural things, any piece of the environment, with our associations to it, thereby con-structing an identity additional to the one generally recog-nized. At heightened moments anything can gain the aura of a personage. But in art it should not be we who do all the imaginative work in this way. The better we understand art the less of the content we impose, the more becomes com-municated. In adopting an aesthetic viewpoint—this, indeed, is a necessary contribution on our part—which we have learned from studying many works of art, we discover that to a considerable extent our attention is confined to the rela-tionship of formal attributes and of their image-creating relevance to the subject matter. The work of art should be to some extent a strait-jacket in regard to the eventual images that it is most likely to induce. Obviously any mode of feeling can be communicated by art, perhaps even by abstract art. Nevertheless the personification of that message in the terms of aesthetic form constructs a simulacrum, a presence that qualifies the image of the paramount feeling expressed. That feeling takes to itself as a crowning attribute more general images of experience. Form, then, ultimately constructs an image or figure of which, in art, the expression of particular feeling avails itself. A simple instance lies with Bonnard, with the shape of hats in his time that approximated to the shape of the head and indeed of the breast. He seems to co-ordinate experience largely through an unenvious and loving attitude to this form. He is equally interested in a concave rounded shape. Again, when we know well an artist and his work we may feel that among the characteristic forms he makes some

48

at least are tied to an image of his own physique or of a personal aspect in his physical responses. This also would be an instance of form as an agent which, through the means of the artist's personality as an evident first step in substantiation, allows him to construct from psychical and emotional as well as physical concatenations a thing that we tend to read as we read a face. A face records more experience than its attention at the moment we look at it.

Perhaps all we demand of a work of art is that it should be as a face in this sense. But form in the widest sense of all, as the attempted organization that rules every experience, must obviously give rise to a strong and compelling imagery so generalized that it can hardly be absent from a consciousness in working order though ordinarily present in nothing like the aesthetic strength, since were it otherwise refreshment and encouragement that we gain from art would not be necessary. Form must possess the character of a compelling apparition, and it is easy to realize that it is the icon of co-ordination.

Integration or co-ordination of what? it will be asked. Some aspect, I have argued elsewhere, of the integration of experience, of the self, with which is bound up the integrity of other people and of other things as separate, even though the artist has identified an aspect of himself with the object, has transfixed the object with his own compulsion, though not to the extent of utterly overpowering its otherness. These perceptions of relationship that are the basis of a minimum sanity demand reinforcement. Outwardness, a physical or concrete adaptation of relationship, spells out enlargement, means certainty.

It must appear a strange suggestion that art is in any way bent upon constructing an image for sanity, however minimal, in view of the wild unbalanced strains of feeling that have so often been inseparably employed in making this image. But surely if art allows not only the extremity of expressiveness but the most conclusive mode, if it constructs of expressiveness an enduring thing, that mode must incorporate an element to transcend or ennoble a particular expressiveness of which otherwise we should soon tire. We are encouraged to experience a many-sided apprehension in art. Expressiveness —it may be infantile—becomes valuable in evolving the mature embrace by form.

In the case of abstract art we are sometimes told by the artist—and it is very understandable—that we entirely mistake his work if we insist it expresses this or that. It is itself, the artist says, it does not stand for, it does not express, anything: it is not meant to suggest associations. I think he is right in the sense he means it. He is providing us, however, in his work with an experience of spatial relationships. Now it is obvious that no experience is entirely isolated, or else it is traumatic. The experience communicated by the abstract artist, on the contrary, invites comparison with other experiences and, to some extent certainly, will point to common ground with a particular aspect of visual experience in the first place or of the relationship between experiences. Abstract art would otherwise be virtually meaningless. Hence we have here an amalgam of meaning conveyed by material that transmits an image not only optical but for the mind or memory as well; unique for the eye but generalized for the mind. Here too the form constrains us to an image, and it is not merely one of our choosing.

Aesthetic experience can be defined as the opposite, indeed often as a palliative, of traumatic experience. But I am not going to try to probe the conditions of being of which this aspect of form is the symbol. I have attempted this elsewhere, as I have said. Some of the preliminaries are straightforward —for instance, the connection with the body-image. I shall partly be confining myself to this aspect.

I have often before referred to the rough-and-smooth values in building, in architecture, that are carried over into the other visual arts and, indeed, into the textures, as we have to call them, of concerted sound. Why otherwise are we forced to speak of texture to describe appositions of instrumental sound? In truth, we cannot but speak of the surface of any work of art, and equally of shape and volume, of the articulated body, metaphors by which we assert the dynamic effect of its impression and the self-completeness. Formal values vivify such images; the inevitable metaphors derive from inevitable images that accompany our apprehension of the formal qualities. In the fifteenth-century courtyard of the palace at Urbino designed by Luciano Laurana, in my opinion one of the greatest masterpieces of architecture, we surely see the same thing, a justice and fairness in the smoothness of the pilasters on the brick wall. The strength of this wall is measured by the eloquence of its apertures and by the open arcade beneath. Each plain yet costly member of this building has the value of a limb: in the co-ordination of the contrasting materials there is equal care for each: together they make stillness that, as it were, breathes.

One must agree to a generalized and meaningful content in the relationships of the Soto construction and in the Laurana courtyard. But are they characteristic works of art, that is to say so characteristic that they can be used to illustrate a content available in all art? What of the agony, violence, irregularity, flippancy even, that appear to be inevitable in some art today, or the restlessness, the explosive disruptiveness that is also common to much of the art of the past?

I have said that the generalized content of form, an element of co-ordination as well as of allusiveness, not only does not inhibit but makes an enduring thing or body of any kind of expressiveness however extreme. When, as has been common in this country, we use the term 'expressionist' in a pejorative sense, we mean that unmistakable expressiveness figures in this or that work but is by no means richly integrated throughout the formal relationships on view, and that therefore the effect is transitory rather than enduring. It encompasses no more than one or two notes. From Picasso's *Three Dancers* at the Tate, on the contrary, we derive a shattering image that coheres. It merits a lot of study. In the Tate *Annual Report* for 1964-5 there is a remarkable analysis, I think the best account I have read of a modern painting. It shows that every piece of the canvas is emotive, contributing to the whole, and even that there are resumed two of the most expressive themes in the iconography of Christian art. I need not go into it: in fact to do so would not help my purpose at this moment, the purpose of reminding you that we are instantaneously convinced by this agitated scene, though it is disruptive and difficult to understand. But we see that every line and tone and division helps in the setting up of various relationships across and down the face of the canvas. In front of an insistently imaginative painting this tends to convince us that an emotive or poetic whole is there expressed, since the expressiveness is transmitted by a rich language of form. Were it not so it would be a bad picture. The echoes and relationships make expressiveness ring, reverberate. Poetry may be plain and simple: the reverberations, even so, are many. Similarly with the nude in visual art. Form encourages further meaning because it is itself the container of a sum of meanings; the nude has already a variety of intense meanings, even apart from art and apart from the connection between the body and form.

In the mechanism of this reverberation prime objects, however transmuted, will figure. Parts of the body and the body itself are prime objects instituting relationships at the root of subsequent relationships of every kind. Our awareness of the violent distortions and the formal elaboration of the breast in the Picasso *Three Dancers*, leading to a round void in the middle of the dancer on the left, illustrates that the body is an object we are likely to follow keenly in transmutations imposed by the artist. I am eager to point out that an ideal

52

Madonna by Raphael is no traitor to this wide connective-
ness.

But first Cézanne and the other very great painting that we
have of late welcomed to this country, *Les Baigneuses*, in the
National Gallery. At first sight these figures could suggest a
quorum of naked tramps camped on top of railway carriages
as the landscape roars by from left to right; except, of course,
that studied, monumental, they altogether refuse the character of silhouettes. They absorb, and in absorbing rule, the
environment. Beyond the long seal-like woman who regards
the depths of the background, the standing, studious, twin-like
girls with backs to us lean across towards the trees and clouds
as if to be those upright trees. All the same the stretching
across the picture plane is more intense, the stretching of
these governing bodies that now seem poised on the easy
rack of a level moving staircase. But movement to the left is
blocked by the striding figures on that side, and since movement is braked at the other end as well it is as if shunted
trucks were held between two engines. The tall, contemplative
figure on the further bank remembers for us the stretching
movement that, in effect, has crammed the centre where the
two groups of bathers meet. Rich with dynamic suggestions,
the movements coalesce into a momentary composure so that
even within the crowd there appears to be airiness and space.
It is now that we contemplate the broad back, laid out like a
map, of the sitting woman with black hair on the left. Only in
art, in an image, in a concrete realization of emotional bents,
such powers with their reconciliation are found perfected.

Another image comes to us in terms of the heads of
hair of walnut and stained oak. It speaks to us of the
strength of the trees in those women and of the tawny arena
on which the bodies lie and, by contrast, it includes the
circumambient blue, the knife-like blue day that these nudes
have crowded to inhabit. They feed on the blue, on the distance at which the seal-woman exclaims. The close, clumsy

yet heroic flesh sips the sky. These nudes are blue-consuming objects and blue is the only colour almost entirely absent from all the varieties of nourishment. The dissociation invites us to examine them more for their sculptural value, to grasp the monumentality not only of the group but of the knife-sharp, simplified faces without mouths, the alternations between astounding bulk and summary, distorted sharpness that both underwrite the compositional movements and, from a faceted flatness, heighten the picture plane. The sky too is faceted, spread thick like butter.

The distorted angularity of many shoulders, the insistence upon angle and strength of line, oppose with ferocity a facile mingling of these bodies, in order to rejoin them sharply; with the result that our apprehension of the bulky, answering V shapes is a startled apprehension, as if experienced by means of the extreme flare of a forked lightning flash. Coupled with the contrasting monumentality, this sharpness persists in the impression however long we gaze. Another reconciliation is between the sheet-lightning of the enwrapping towels and the slow swathes of blue daylight that dwell on ochre-tinted flesh and ochre hair and the ochreous strand.

For me the blue embrace is the final impression, withstanding a hurricane-like flattening of the light-toned foliage and a suggestion in the shape of the right-hand bathers' group of a petal-shaped volcanic orifice erupting into a steamy cloud beyond. But the group as a whole does not appear settled or rooted to the ground. The figures almost slide on it. We sense the possibility of fresh forms burrowing up from the ground's lightness to meet the blue embrace. This sense of lightness and fruitfulness balances yet enhances both monumentality and angularity.

The left-hand group is pyramidal; incline of the tree-trunks is an important element of the design, in the arrest and, on the right, in the reversal of movement. But especially in regard to so great and complex a picture I am the more unwilling to speak in the plainer functional terms of composition and design. I prefer to insist that the formal elements not only enrich but enlarge the subject matter. The fact that you do not agree with every image that I have associated with this picture does not invalidate my point. The emotive arrangements carry a number of such interpretations. Form is the container for a sum of meanings while it is from a concatenation of meanings that form is constructed, meanings that have been translated into terms of spatial significance. Without appreciation of spatial value, of empathy with bodies in space, there can be no understanding of the emotive images that form conveys. I believe that there is a nexus of meaning that we all recognize however various our explanations; it is composed from experiences otherwise divergent. The experiences will be largely individual but the power of an integrated communion between trends in concrete or corporeal terms is palpable. Let us agree that the material for creating this nexus is drawn from the artist's experiences and intentions, particularly, of course, his aims in regard to art. There are also broader limitations upon the realization of form without which we have no licence to conceive of art, matters of style, of the moment in the history of art and of the culture it mirrors, the many-sided limitations that are the concern of art history. But here, too, proper understanding depends upon an acceptance that cultural aim has been translated by all art, even sometimes without the help of iconography, into the concrete terms of the senses and within the range of our long memory for sensory experiences wherein traces of the first and primary objects are preserved. One more word about *The Bathers*. Some of the faces particularly are conceived as a series of ledges or blocks, wooden, primitive, strong. The tendency exists throughout Cézanne's development from the seventies. I believe this aspect of his work, especially in the last compositions of Bathers, is the first of his influences upon the evolution of Cubism. This same aspect of his influence is far more obvious upon *Les Demoiselles D'Avignon* and upon all those works that were so soon to forge the easiest of links with Negro sculpture. I cannot help speculating in the most far-fetched manner whether one day it will be possible to claim for *The Bathers* that it is among the first and perhaps the greatest works of a deeply founded cosmopolitan art which was to pre-figure the eventual evolution of a multi-racial society. That would indeed be to specify a very pregnant image implicit in form, the compulsions of which in the Industrial Age had substantiated out of the inner life a compulsion even of a history to be.

No manifestation, particularly psychological manifestation, no behaviour, no ritual, is as foreign as it was. We found a new culture from remnants that remain of our own and possibly from what we have understood of other cultures past and present. If one had to choose to say only one thing about modern art, it would have to be in relation to this, it seems to me, not as a matter of ideas, of rationalizations, but as avid necessity in regard to an externalization of the inner life, deeply qualified, as for an art activity it must be, by the social setting, by the look, by the quality of the external world on which the social setting has been projected.

The controlled tenderness of Bellini's Christian piety, as seen in *The Dead Christ supported by Angels* (National Gallery), embraces an illumined land. That view of the body had come down to him from Attic Greece. Pentelic sanity confronts muted eloquence. The stillness of the candid dead torso dignifies life without separating it from grief. Dead, the body of Christ connects with the living who take into their minds the image of Christ as an ideal body, it is suggested here, as a chest in part, smooth, sloping, elephantine in wisdom; breathing, it seems, a warm silence. More generally we are offered images of life and death, deft angels and the mortified head of the corpse. The habit of bodies, whether sensitive

56

or dead, is disclosed once more: we are told that in the variety of meanings to which it points a body is as expressive as a face. The partial nude always conveys the sense of disclosure: it is appropriate here to the Christian meaning. At the same time the angels perform a slow gentle wrapping of the corpse.

Many characteristics of flesh are suggested by this delineation, but only one characteristic is omni-present to which other delineations are subordinate: shape against a background. The spaces thus contrived are roughly triangles. The angels' heads both echo and vary Christ's head, the cylinders of their arms the corpse's arms. The element of geometry or of reduplication is an armature, the aesthetic armature, to which our feelings, as if they too could be solid things, as if they could be clay, cling; that is to say our feelings of contact, our meeting with a separated object or with ourselves now encouraged to separate from the splitting of ourselves. We feel in ourselves the tautness of the angels' feathered wings, the wrinkled clinging sleeve, the arm covering in the making for the corpse below those wings. We feel in us the corpse's beautiful listless hands. Christ's right arm droops but it is half-supported by a ledge on which the fingers bend, and by the angels' enwrapping grip. That demonstration of gravity serves less the effect of momentum than of poise, so nearly compounded of compensations as to be rest.

How often is this the effect upon us of the Old Masters, particularly of paintings with nudes. In my own mind I revisit early years abroad, the sense of discovery in many galleries, the predominant effect of the pictures in relation to the discomfiture of loneliness. Art meant oasis for the body as well as for the mind but also a ritual that affirmed unalterable contact, on the whole in a fully adult sense, rescued from the excess that had obscured or depleted an embrace.

Rembrandt's *Belshazzar's Feast* in the National Gallery is far from conveying this involucre of Pentelic marble; on the

57

contrary, it shows human beings with the incorrigible character of scored, used pots. A darker conception of the body assumes a vivid clay. Hence Belshazzar's imposing pallor even though he suggests a richly feathered hen or turkey amid a treasury of filth, though the quilted magisterial stomach mounts to a plucked neck and head. Leaden with the threads of gold and silver, turban and diadem reiterate the blindness of heaped matter as does the great weighted see-saw of Belshazzar's outstretched arms. The woman recoiling on the right who spills from a cup herself suggests a rounded, stoppered vessel. The clattering gold, like all treasure, has its threat or is threatened. Amid the fur of light upon the wall incomprehensible letters speak out the traumatic counterpart sometimes associated with these bodily products.

I believe that strong feelings of such a kind, or feelings derived from them, possessed Rembrandt; they are one root of his power; and that otherwise he could not so magnificently have imposed the weighty articulation, for instance, of Belshazzar's right hand.

Many of us find Rembrandt to be the greatest of artists, I think because no artist approaches him in projecting the feel I have spoken of, the feel of presences not only substantiated from observation in the outside world but substantiated equally from the hazy presences in the mind. We are aware of a lineage for his every face far beyond the range of iconographic study. These presences are charged, weighty, condensed from the light and from the dark literally and metaphorically, with a finer drama than the apparition of writing on a wall. They are compendia, bodies that manifest the history of their growth: each speck gives power to an opaque fellow. In a very remarkable book about Soutine, just published, Andrew Forge has written of Rembrandt in similar strain. He has this sentence: 'This is his (Rembrandt's) measure, that his architecture is as ambitious as his material is earthy.'

We are sometimes shown in contemporary art heads as helmets. The projecting plane for forehead and nose folds sharply back. How beautiful the helmet-shape in Raphael's [2] *Madonna of the Tower* (National Gallery) of the shoulder's overdress, the suave shoulder bone above it, the rounded neck, the geometrical expanse of face and head turned towards us! Were the helmet-shape armour, it would not allow smoothness to the firm skin, nor stillness above the straining child. The shoulder's rotund slope is developed across the picture by the child's undeveloped, trusting arm; we give a more than usual value to the continuation since we are even ready to connect the discontinued in view of the felicity to each other of helmet-shoulder and Virgin's head, an unarmed Athene. There is added poignancy too in the more rounded head of the child pressed and tilted away by the contact with his mother's cheek, and in her hand that comes round the child's middle and in the other hand that holds his foot. The curved line of the Virgin's cheek against the darkness where the child's temple flares—there is much triangularity as well as roundness in the composition—possesses an eloquence of eyelids. The faint encircling veil that depends from the summit of the Virgin's head reinforces the group's monumentality, not least this gravity of warmth and love.

The picture's ruined state makes one wonder the more at the beauty of the whole, at the regularity of the head, at the Michelangelesque *contrapposto* of the sitting body; at the cliff-like excesses and irregular caverns of the voluminous outer garment that consorts with the smooth flat hair, with the calm landscape and the simplicity of the Virgin's face.

In considering thus the composition's sentiment we touch other states of mind as bodily things, even an account of acceptance and rejection, since visual art works pre-eminently with contrast, with relief and background, with light and dark, with emphasis and its curb, with the play of opposing surfaces and degrees of volume. The ceaseless metaphors of language are physical and physiological. We stretch them painfully in pure speculation. Art corrects abstraction. Even the good and the bad mirror their physiological derivation: what is physiologically good gives rise to what is bad when we are deprived of it or when—and that is always—it is the object of our envious selves. The language of disdain, hatred, and rejection discovers the utmost denunciation in the terms of putrefaction. We speak of the currents of our feeling as dismembered, split, or perhaps they are not crippled.

Abstractions tend to become presences in dreams. Parents from the earliest times and other people are presences within, and when the self projects part of itself it projects an object. There are images in our lives to which we hold tenaciously; we rediscover them in their variants. These are embodied operations that allow to art a universal language.

What great demands, then, we make of the artist, and how supremely great is the great artist! This painting satisfies as a reconstruction of mother and child. The sentiment is forthright but with it the artist has forged wider attachments that continue to fascinate our reflective selves. They helped the artist to typify his theme in accordance, of course, with the development and state of art at that moment, in accordance with the influence upon him from his art and from his culture, not to mention requirements of the patron. The culture served by Raphael obtained expression in his image of the subject matter that was determined also by much that he attributed to relationships in space. Or these last, it could be said, were the vehicle of a particular Christian sentiment. It makes no difference to my point which way round the matter is put. And my point is that we have not only the image of Virgin and Child presented in accordance with Italian iconography and pictorial style of the early sixteenth century but also the sixteenth-century iconography or pictorial style of relationship in man's inner world in the concrete terms of space applied to, and modified by—even inspired by—the subject of mother and child.

I can think of no other Old Master landscape painting beside Hobbema's *Brederode Castle* (National Gallery), unless it be the *Amsterdam Herring Tower*, also by Hobbema, also in the National Gallery, and equally jewel-like in colour, that gives as strongly an impression to be discovered in most landscape, namely the impression that though one is scanning the open, the distant, at the same time one is imaginatively attending to an interior scene, an aspect of the inner life. This castle landscape, stepped from blue to red, to the dark bank, to the pink ruin and to the incontinent clouds like the disordered roof of a cave, is yet so softly and closely organized that the castle may seem to have the function of a high altar at a cathedral's end or, more simply, to suggest the centre of a cupped flower. The central mass is echoed by the forms of the bank and trees in the left foreground though they are much darker, larger, flowing or ragged. The Amsterdam townscape is somewhat similarly composed in this respect. I suggest that as well as looking on the outside world we are looking at personable figures ensconced in the mind that exert intermittent influence on the pliable forefront of our attention.

In a changing landscape the pink buildings are these static personages, or rather the good personages who have survived every attack, whom we wish would never surrender their places; whom we want to be static even as ruins. They are shown here as receivers of the passing light and of the seasons. But there is sap in the trees, in bushes and grasses: the dark river, like the blood, like circumstance, flows in a circular channel: the river birds are community members, while the buildings are bare of all except simple structure; apertures, buttress, walls with an accretion only of fern.

Viewed as an image of mind and body the painting shows the flesh, with the forces that animate and those to which it is subject, as divided, as mingled in new combinations. Yet

61

owing to the compelling insinuation of tone and colour a totality emerges from these divisions and admixtures, having learned from them an intimacy or warmth that now serves the central structure and its surroundings; a totality that the eye reassembles and communicates at each look.

Of such kind, I believe, is the reckoning demanded of us by the just accountancy of great paintings in regard not only to masses but to the use of paint, to tone and colour relationships, to the representation of texture, movement, light. An image of building as generic structure, rich in itself yet palpitating with the cursive endowments also of the surrounding world with which it abides in relation, has been an inherent theme of our culture and of our art since classical times, to which even this seventeenth-century northern landscape must be referred. Building has figured in nearly all our landscape painting up to the middle of the last century when architecture for the first time ceased to epitomize the co-ordination of the body and thereby the integration of the ego, of the person or the mind. Yet while the old theme was notably exploited by Corot at times, he and those who accompanied and followed him have continued to provide through the texture of their paint, or through other insistence on the picture plane, many of those surface values that an environment of architecture once had lavished.

I end on a favourite note after developing the argument with the help of a minute fragment from the variety of art. Nothing, for instance, from outside Europe. I have offered images that are, at best, sometimes appropriate to the formal elements of the pictures described—in association of course with their subject matter. Once more, as a last word, I ask you not to identify these images, these derivatives, with what I have called the 'image in form', that is, where I have spoken of it as a generalized happening implicit in all the differing manifestations a few of which I have tried to interpret. The proof of this generalized happening that seeks to dispel chaos does not rely only on such speculative, subjective assertions. Now the chaotic is at best only just behind all of us, and we discover certainty largely by a massive projection of ourselves on to the external world which we then reabsorb. This generalized happening, it seems to me, has direct bearing on the correspondence between sensuous arrangements in the outside world and the conscious—I have spoken so far only of the less conscious—images we sometimes form of our mental processes. For we find in our reflective states that simple emotions or complicated wishes both to have and not to have something, states of tension, capacities of the mind and so on, have themselves implanted as we contemplated them a residue of spatial imagery that we can watch; intersecting lines of conflict; stubborn, seemingly material, obstacles; rhythms and intervals that correspond with the order and tempo of events, the punctuation of time; spatial images, these, of sensation and a sum of experience which, when transposed into an art activity with material, provides the means of a concrete language whose expressiveness depends upon firm links with the continuous inner images substantiating and ordering complicated experiences of the body and of the mind; but hitherto substantiating in an unfixed manner. And so we see why painting, for instance, is primarily concerned with projecting the third dimension, why we value so highly the whole range of disposition from shapes that loom to those exactly disposed, the obstinate suggestion of volume or of depth magnificently achieved in all my examples, even the Soto [3]. In any visual construction we require not only provocative nouns, so to speak, of insistent shape but equally interconnection, the action one upon another, analogous to the role of verbs upon which a statement depends. Since the glimmering nouns behind the concrete forms are strongly comprehensive yet ambiguous, the fixing verb-function of composition is likely to be many-sided. Moreover all the statements of whatever kind in a picture tend to be very closely interconnected since they are apprehended together, since their contents are simultaneously revealed. A great painter like Seurat is able to extract the utmost significance for his compositions from the slightest variation in a few dominant forms or directions.

An easy thing remains to be said; a *caveat*. Pictures are not problems. Nothing I have put forward, even supposing it to be correct, alters the fact that the Hobbema is a landscape painting wherein the artist communicates his pleasure, his record of a natural scene containing castle, ducks, trees, and people. This topographical value is the only value admitted by some who, for whatever reason, are entirely impervious to art. We should be in little better case than they if the considerations I have advanced, instead of supplementing or interpreting that immediate aspect of the matter, undermined it.

NOTES

1. Adapted from a lecture given with slides.
2. Ascribed to Raphael. One can say with certainty that the major design is his.
3. Cf. Professor Wollheim's inaugural lecture of 1964, where he argued that a mark made on paper causes not only configuration but representation in nearly all cases. *On Drawing an Object*, Richard Wollheim (London, H. K. Lewis, 1965).

Printed and bound by CPI Group (UK) Ltd, Croydon, CR0 4YY

01/11/2024

01782629-0012